MW00677036

The Superwoman Complex

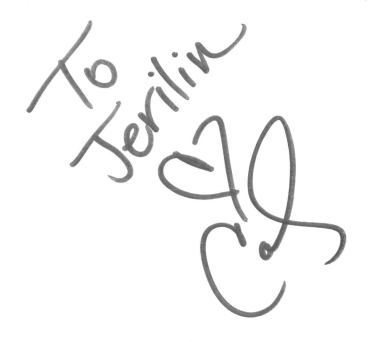

The Superwoman Complex:

A Follow-Up Visit

By C. Nicole Swiner, MD

Copyright © 2016 Swiner Publishing Company

All rights reserved.

ISBN : 978-0-9863702-1-2
ISBN :

Table of Contents

Prelude   vii

Foreword   ix

Thanks and Gratitude   xi

Introduction   xiii

Chapter 1: Love What You Do, and Do What You Love   1

Chapter 2: Loving Relationships and #Tribes   10

Chapter 3: Living a Joyful Life...On Purpose   23

Chapter 4: Time for a Check-Up   30

Chapter 5: The Sleepy-Mama Syndrome   37

Chapter 6: The Curvy Controversy   44

Chapter 7: Pack Light   50

Chapter 8: Don't Rock the Boat   55

Chapter 9: The SuperMAN Complex   61

Chapter 10: Holiday Stress   68

Chapter 11: New Year, New You   74

References   80

The Superwoman Complex: A Follow-Up Visit

Prelude

Everyone's financial, household or job setup is different, so some of the changes I made may not be feasible for you. That's okay! The goal is to start thinking about what changes you can make. Figure out what best works for you. Start with more simple remedies. If your job is awesome but the commute is a nightmare, look into a car/vanpool option or even better, talk to your employer about teleworking one or two days per week. If you love your profession but certain aspects are taking a toll on you, consider how to do it differently.

For example, if you're a teacher, consider leading a homeschool group for children in your church or subdivision, working as an education consultant or doing both. If you're totally unhappy as an engineer, begin thinking about what you are happy doing and how you may be able to make a living doing it. These decisions may involve going back to school and/or taking an entrepreneurial leap of faith, but considering the amount of time we spend working, we should spend it doing something that doesn't leave us perpetually stressed. It's important to note that none of this will happen overnight. It may take a year (or three or four), but you have to start somewhere and that's now!

Let's pick up where we left off with the first book. Let's continue to learn.... how to avoid the Superwoman Complex. Enjoy.

Foreword

Perhaps there's no better medicine than the loving, witty, and humorous advice shared between good girlfriends. Dr. Nicole Price Swiner is that comforting voice on the other end of the phone line, administering a healthy dose of healing and hope. As if standing on the sideline of a marathon, she cheers for her readers and encourages them to abandon the pressure to be perfect. Instead she writes a prescription for rest and more importantly, fun while juggling the demands of family life. Debunking the Superwoman myth is definitely worth a follow-up visit. Page by page, the good doctor is a reliable and supportive sister- friend who reminds us we can be super and women.

Tamara Gibbs
Author of Single Serving for Single Women
Client of Swiner Publishing Company

The best care always includes fantastic follow-up! That's just what Dr. Swiner/Docswiner delivers in this timely sequel to "How To Avoid The Superwoman Complex". You'll immediately recognize the caring voice backed by the wealth of knowledge and matter-of-fact wit that is her signature style.

The follow-up visit does more than just check to see how you've been doing with your new tips and habits. Dr. Swiner is back with even more advice that puts her medical knowledge right in your hands in everyday words and exercises to get you moving. She explores a range of key topics like how your relationship is affecting your health, the subtle things at work that could be draining your happiness, and simple changes to make sure you're living your best life.

My favorite part of this book is that you can feel Docswiner's passion for medicine, zeal for life, and love for her patients coming through in every word. It's inspiring. It makes me want to be healthier to do more for longer with the ones I love. I trust it will do the same for you.

Dr. Mani Saint-Victor, "Break The Cage", MD
Co-founder of "Thinking About Quitting Medicine"

Thanks and Gratitude

This past year has been phenomenal. I truly couldn't have pursued my passion without the encouragement and love from the following folks:

My Lord and Savior, Jesus Christ
My family-The love of my life, Ric, and our 2 beautiful girls
My Daddy, Mama (rest in Heaven), brother Reginald and sis-in-law (and Editor-In-Chief of both books) Nicole
My Swiner family
My #Durm (Durham, NC) music, arts and think tank tribe (You know who you are)
My clinic-Durham Family Medicine-for putting up with my multitasking and rescheduling
My patients-for also putting up with the above
My assistant, Amy Maynard-for all of your hard work and being Jane on the spot
I-Cubed Agency for help and great advice
For supportive groups-WERock Atlanta, Mocha Medicine, PMG, Delta Sigma Theta Sorority, Inc., No Fear of Oklahoma City, MUSC, UNC

Thanks and Gratitude

My church-Union Baptist Church and Pastor and First
Lady Hammond
My home church-Truth and Fellowship Ministry
and Pastor Briggs
Any and all organizations that have invited me to speak this
past year
And last but not least....all of you who have purchased this
book.
I thank you.
-Docswiner

Introduction

The Superwoman Complex: A Follow- Up Visit

Hello again! Funny to think it's been less than a year since I sat down and decided to pen the first book. Since March 2015, it's been a whirlwind! I, along with my family and friends, have worked, and shared, and called, and emailed and begged for this "book tour" of mine to happen. It's been going well, with TV appearances, book signings and speaking engagements a couple of times a month. And during most of it, the next question has usually been, "So, when's the next one coming out?" It's almost similar to when you first get married. Before you can even enjoy the first moment, folks begin asking the question, "So, when are you going to have kids", allowing no time to breathe.

Well, here we go!

The Superwoman Complex: A Follow-Up Visit

I named this one the "Follow-Up Visit," because I'm a doctor, and doctors live for the follow-ups. But I also wanted to bring readers back in to delve deeper into the topics I mentioned in the first book. People that I met who read the book often said they wanted to know more about the this complex and how to battle it. I almost tricked readers, on purpose, of course, into learning more about important medical topics than they probably wanted to, and then teased a little about what to do about the Superwoman Complex. So, that's what I intend to do. Give you more.

I hope you enjoyed the first book, and I hope you enjoy this one as well. Let's delve in together, once more, and come out the other side a more settled, calm and relaxed Us.

While I was laying down the foundation for this book, the Charleston 9 tragedy occurred. If you had your head stuck in the sand during this time, it was a sad display of racism that befell 9 innocent victims at Mother Emanuel AME church in downtown Charleston, my hometown. A shooter went into the church, sat with the congregation that welcomed him into their worship service, and ended their lives all in the name of racism. I've been feeling depressed and saddened ever since, and I've tried to hold my tongue as much as possible in an effort to not offend and also to avoid the sadness. But since I have a platform...the most disheartening thing about it is even while being peaceful and serving our God, we can be gunned down for no reason what-so-ever. I pray for our nation, our world and my children who have to endure this hatred that we worked for decades, that civil rights soldiers like Dr. King, Jr., worked for decades to eradicate. I love this country, but I'm very disappointed in all of us for fostering this kind of behavior and allowing this to happen. We all played a part in allowing that racist comment to come out of the mouth of our friend as we laughed along or stood idly by....or by turning the other cheek, while a fellow citizen was being discriminated against...or even by allowing a stereotype of the culture we represent to go unchecked. We all must do better. If for no one else's sake, do it for my children's sake.

On a lighter note, this (no) superwoman movement has been enlightening and exhilarating. I had no idea how many women shared the same struggles and challenges—both inner and external—that force us to feel "some type of way" about what being a woman means. I'm glad that we're talking about it more, and being more open about needing guidance and good advice to help us through the phases of being wives, working women (or stay at home Moms,) and mothers. Let's keep talking.

The Superwoman Complex: A Follow-Up Visit

One idea that I faced while promoting and talking about the first book was a question of, "Will people think I'm saying it's ok for women to be lazy in a sense?" I even had one husband, jokingly (or at least I think he was joking), ask, "Does this mean my wife will read this and want to stop working?" He clearly wasn't pleased about this idea. I responded by saying no, but what if she would be happier (and as a result, the family would be happier) by her working a little less and decreasing her stress level? Why is that a bad thing? So, let me clarify----this idea is in no way a cop out for women. I never said quit your jobs and sit on your lazy bottoms and do nothing. I'm, in fact, saying the opposite. Be successful, but be happy at the same time. Have your goals, whether they exist at school or at your job, but you may have to do it in phases, or take some time off or change career paths so it works better for you in the long run. Don't burn yourself out. Work and be successful---but stop running yourself ragged.

It's also been interesting encountering women in the community, mostly retired or baby boomers, that say, "Oh, I don't need that book" or "I used to be a Superwoman, but not anymore." They seem to know all the answers. Do you know why? It's because they no longer have the syndrome because they were retired or the kids had grown up and left the house. What a realization that was for me. But, not all of us are there yet. We still have jobs and have kids to raise, and parents to take care of, and career moves to make....so we have a while yet before that euphoria hits.

Now. The BIG question is; how do we do this? Let's turn the page, shall we?

Chapter 1

Love What You Do, & Do What You Love

Imagine burning a candle from both ends.

Once it's gone, it's gone, and there's nothing left for you or anyone else. Anyone on any job can experience burnout, but this is an especially popular topic with doctors these days because many of us are dealing with it in some way. Some doctors are quitting medicine altogether, working less hours, or continuing to work but in an unhappy, unfulfilled space.

When I wrote my first book, "How to Avoid the Superwoman Complex: 12 Ways to Balance Mind, Body & Spirit," I was rounding out my eighth year of working full time as a family doctor. I was having fun seeing patients all day long, but not so much fun managing hours of insurance-related paperwork and phone calls, which is not taught in medical school or residency – doctors learn the ins-and-outs of business once we start working in the real world. So, I had to get creative to prevent burn-out.

First, here's a quick review of the last chapter of the first book on what I do (and still do) to stay sane:

1. Marry the right spouse/pick the right partner.
2. Maintain the relationship/continue to date one another.
3. Ask for help...a lot.
4. Hire help.
5. Exercise.
6. Pray and meditate.
7. Pamper yourself.
8. Bring them to you/use mobile services.
9. Go to sleep.
10. Get therapy.
11. Have an occasional cocktail.
12. Take a vacation or mental health day.
13. Have girls'/guys' night out.

What I did over the last year was try to focus on what I enjoy most – meeting new people, community service, women's health, pediatrics, stress reduction and relaxation. I'd been writing and sharing ideas via social media for some time, and decided to fashion those ideas into a book. I also began leading group visits with patients, doing several well-child or weight loss visits at one time, an interesting twist to the typical doctor's appointment, which allowed my patients to interact more and glean from each other. Because I have control over my schedule, I cut my afternoons, giving me more time to spend with my family. Eventually, I began taking every other Friday off for longer weekends twice a month.

The question is how can we do this for everyone? In Book 1, we discussed taking a day for a mental health break. Why work and earn these vacation days, if you don't take advantage of them? And taking a vacation day doesn't necessarily mean spending loads of money to go to the Caribbean, either. It could mean taking a Friday and a Monday off for an extra long "staycation" at home. I love a couple of quiet days at home, when the girls are in school, so I can clean up a bit, watch TV by myself or take a nap. How lovely!

Last year, I had the honor of speaking to some family medicine residents and medical students at the University of Maryland-Baltimore. We spent time connecting and reviewing how difficult and challenging these years can be, but not to fret. As one of my favorite gospel songs says, "Trouble don't last always." However, it doesn't end with graduating and finishing med school or residency. Real life, and work, follow. I shared a lesson, entitled "What I Wish I Knew……" to enlighten them on how I view things since I graduated from residency 8 years ago. I was asked the following questions—

How did you choose the life you lead and was it a conscious decision?

I think I was encouraged as a child to choose a career and lifestyle that were going to be a positive one and an enjoyable one. My faith in God and my parents' focus on our faith early on definitely helped the decision to live the life I live. I'd like to think it was a mixture of nature and nurture in choosing the life that I now lead… and favor from Jesus!

Why did you select your area of medical expertise? And what is the most challenging aspect of working in the healthcare field?

I always thought I would have been a pediatrician from the time I was in high school. After getting into med school, however, and being exposed to different fields, I learned I had a love of OB-gyn medicine. The lifestyle, stress, and hours OBs kept, were deterrents. At the end of my 3rd year of med school, I did my Family Medicine rotation and had my "Aha" moment. It was the perfect mix of seeing babies and their families, from the cradle to the grave, along with the option of delivering babies, if I wanted to. I haven't turned back yet.

The most challenging aspect is the burden of taking care of those who don't want to take care of themselves. Doctors, the good ones, often care more about patients than they do about themselves. It's very frustrating, also, to be forced to have to see patients with extremely complicated medical histories in 15-20 minutes in order to meet standards and see as many patients as possible to make ends meet. This is why many doctors are getting out of medicine nowadays.

What has been your greatest obstacle in life and how do/ did you navigate it?
Losing my mother about 8 years ago, and working through my Faith and therapy to heal from it.

What has been your greatest life lesson learned to date?
To learn to be happy and joyful in the face of adversity and challenges. It's an ongoing process.

What is your best advice on how to live a graceful life?
Pray, rest, laugh and love often.

With that, I'll add this: If you hate your job, change it. Shorten or change your work schedule. Ask for a promotion or demotion to a different department. Ask for a change of duties or responsibilities. Or get another job or change careers. Are these changes always easy? Nope. But, is it true that it may be worth your sanity? Absolutely. If you can't leave your job right now, how about creating a "side-hustle;" a "side-gig," if you will?

This is defined as a hobby that becomes an activity from which you can make money. You may have a degree in medicine, but you've always also loved to write, or make clothes, or speak, or flip houses. So, why not turn that into an actual business? Talk to an accountant to do paper work or you (it's a huge tax write-off, too) and make it real. You can start just doing it on your days off or the weekends. if you're really successful, maybe it becomes your real gig. It could save your sanity as well, because it'll allow you to do more things you love and are passionate about—like I am now.

Review Questions:

1. Am I truly happy working my current job? If not, why?

2. What can I realistically change about my current situation?

3. Could I work different hours? In a different career or department?

4. Is this what I envisioned I'd be doing when I was little?

Notes: _____

_____

_____

_____

_____

_____

_____

_____

_____

_____

_____

_____

_____

_____

_____

_____

_____

_____

_____

_____

_____

_____

_____

_____

_____

_____

_____

_____

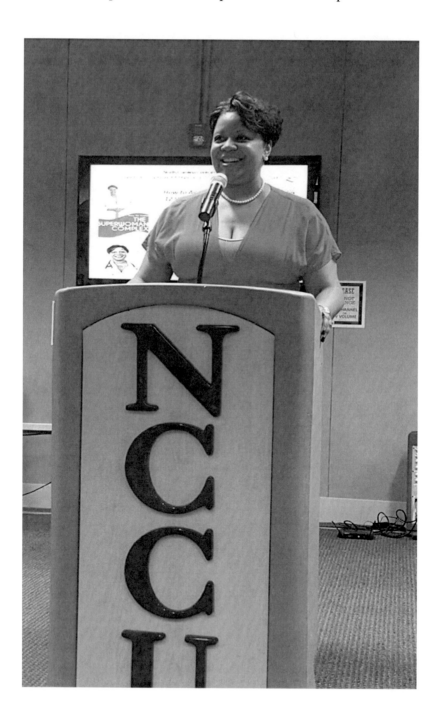

Chapter 2

Loving Relationships and #Tribes

If I could, I'd dedicate this entire book to my husband, Mr. Swiner. If you're close to us or on social media, you probably get tired of me talking about how wonderful of a man he is and about how supportive he's been of this new side-gig of mine. We try to keep our love brewing by having date nights often and paying good attention to each other. Some may think that sharing love on social media jinxes a good relationship. I think that's silly. Don't overdo it, though. No one wants constantly see you kissing and hugging all the time, but occasional "I love you, honey" on Facebook is sweet ☺.

I posted a broadcast on Periscope ™ (a free app that allows live broadcasts and comments) entitled "Friday night shout outs and shoulder pain!" The most important part of it was explaining what Friday night shout outs are to everyone. It's a game that my husband and I created for one another early on in our relationship. We figured, in most relationships, we are bogged down by daily drama, work, stress...you name it. However, your loved one always likes to hear sweet nothings from you to sweeten up your relationship, so why not set out a specific day of the week, every week, to make sure you let them know why you appreciate them. This is good for the 'good feeling' hormones, like your endorphins and your adrenaline, to get things moving, if you know what I mean! It can be as simple as, "Thanks for taking out the trash, Honey;" or "Thanks for buying me a new car," if you're that lucky, but remind your spouse how much you need and appreciate them. My husband, who I consider to be a bit of a love expert himself, always tells me how much a man needs to feel needed and appreciated on a regular basis. It's usually their 'love language,' if you are familiar with that book. So, why not set aside that day, where you are speaking positive things into and about your relationship, to make sure it remains happy.

We all know what an unhealthy and unfulfilling relationship can do to our health, with all the stress that it brings. So, hopefully you have chosen a worthy and deserving partner. If not, changes may need to be made. It's okay to let someone go, if you know that the both of you can be happier either alone or with someone else. Don't stay in an unhealthy or toxic relationship for any reason, and that includes for the children. Children can tell when things are tense and sad in a relationship, and that does not help them to form healthy loving relationships when they grow older, so spare everyone and move on two different environments that will help everyone to be happy. We all know what stress does to the body by now, especially if you have read my book, because I see it on a daily basis as a family doc.

High blood pressure, migraine headaches, constant tension and muscle pain can all be negative effects that we carry around and not even realize are affected by things going on in our lives. Horrible relationships contribute to the Superwoman Complex, and staying in them makes it even worse. However, ending horrible relationships and fostering positive ones defeat the Complex. You don't have to stay in it, just because you feel guilty for leaving or "just for the kids." Plenty of psychologists and psychiatrists will tell you it's more harmful to your and your childrens' mental health to stay in an unhealthy and unsafe marriage environment. So take note, and then do something about it.

This year, Beyonce's #Lemonade album was released. I'm not going to say Bey prompted this next entry, but whatever... ☺ (yes, I'm a fan.)

I have a dear friend who is currently going through a horrible divorce. She is a wonderful lady, phenomenal Mom of 3, and is well-accomplished. I'm worried about her. I, unfortunately, have many friends who have had heart break in relationships, and who are finding their way back to baseline. I thought about them today and what it feels like to establish the "new normal."

I thought about my friend dealing with the drama of dropping her kids off to a condescending, angry ex and waiting for him to pick up the phone at their court allotted Facetime to talk to her kids and say good night. I am overwhelmed with anger when I try to put myself in her shoes and imagine what I'd be feeling.

What I want to say to those women today is, it'll be ok. It hurts now and the tears will fall today, but "trouble don't last always." It's ok to cry for a while, and hate your ex, and feel lonely but know that you are loved and thought about and cared for. Lean on your girlfriends and family to pull you out of the hole. Practice self-care as you know you should. Seek therapy and counseling for you and your children if you need it.

The break-up is likely not all your fault. It takes two to both start and end a relationship. Don't blame yourself for the rest of your life. Learn from the mistakes, mourn the loss (for a short time), and pick yourself back up. You are not your failed relationship. You're more than that.

See this as a REFRESH button, a fresh start. You get to establish the new normal the way YOU want to do it. Sure, it'll be hard at first, but you'll adjust. There will be another love. Be patient. Be careful, but not fearful to love another. Don't carry your baggage with you to the next thing. Know that I'm thinking of you today. Take care.

Now, as far as friendships are concerned...Drake said "No New Friends," but I beg to differ. I completely agree with loving and keeping your old friends, but over this year, I can't express enough how blessed we've been to have met some of the most creative, compelling, inspiring, collaborating folks. They have motivated me to think outside the box and reach goals I'd never thought of. So, yes to both old AND new friends.

As you age, your friend circle generally gets smaller. However, it still remains important to be open to gaining some newbies that encourage you to grow. They support and help you dream the dreams and put them in to action. That's the real definition of #tribe. Drake should change that to "No lame friends." It's important to foster positive friendships. I think 'woman' is a verb. As I've looked around at some of the incredible women in my environment and life, I've been awe-inspired by the examples of Moms, wives, entrepreneurs and single ladies I have. I wanted to touch on the wonderful support and cheerleading I receive from many of them, both near and far.

One of my pet peeves is seeing and hearing women tear other women down. I hear and see it on social media often. Oftentimes, we're super critical of one another and make each other feel guilty for doing the things we do or don't do well. We fat shame and body shame each other and discuss how NOT to trust one another.

Fortunately, I'm part of some groups, online and in real life, such as Delta Sigma Theta Sorority, Inc; EmpowHER; Mocha Medicine; PMG (Physician/Mommy group); that always serve as a sounding board for various issues that may stress me out. I have girlfriends and 3 incredible sisters-in-law who care for me, who although we don't talk daily, I know always have my back and are there to help when I need them.

We take care of husband, boyfriend, partner, girlfriend, children, besties, friends, neighbors, pets...and then maybe...ourselves. We cook, clean, prepare the week, plan the calendar, schedule appointments, do the baby's hair, straighten up and hold down a full-time job. We go to school, go to the gym, carpool, pick up, drop off and wipe noses and tears. Wouldn't you be exhausted?

For Women's History Month, I took a picture with some of my friends here in Durham (see picture at end of chapter). If you're a fan of Beyonce' or her sister, Solange, this "formation" will look familiar. Interpret as you will. Why did we take this, you ask? It all began as a silly idea, but then it quickly became a feeling we liked--one of sisterhood; of fun, love and support. All of us live and work in "#durm," (which is how we like to pronounce Durham). All of these women are about their business--all supporting one another. Most were old friends, some meeting for the first time. No hate. All love. No good reason needed. It personified the definition of tribe.

I'm not sure I'd call myself a feminist, but I love the way women "woman." I'm a fan of us and of how we do (or try to do) all of these things for the betterment of others. Just don't forget you in the process. Don't forget you have other sisters in the struggle to help support you. Ask for help. You are not alone, sister.

Review Questions:

1. Is your love relationship a happy AND HEALTHY one?

2. If not, is there anything you and your partner can change about it? (Mind you, I said change about it and not about each other. You can't change people.)

3. If your relationship is unhappy and unhealthy, why are you still there?

4. Are your friendships loving or toxic? Are they equal in give and take? (We both know what the answers to both of these questions should be in the positive. If not, there's a problem.)

Notes: _____

_____

_____

_____

_____

_____

_____

_____

_____

_____

_____

_____

_____

_____

_____

_____

_____

_____

_____

_____

_____

_____

_____

_____

_____

_____

_____

_____

_____

_____

_____

The Superwoman Complex: A Follow-Up Visit

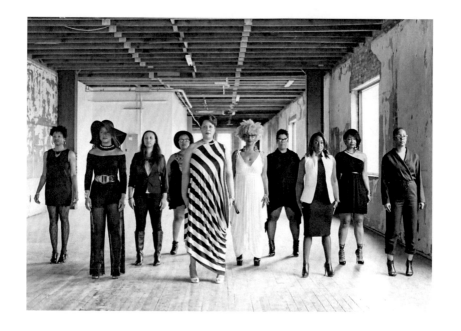

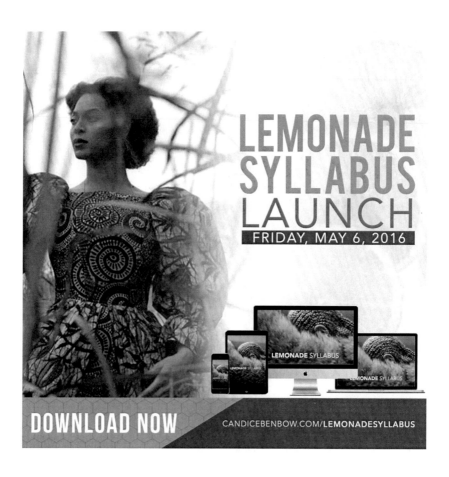

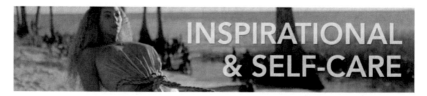

INSPIRATIONAL & SELF-CARE

TITLE	AUTHOR	DATE READ
Can A Sister Get a Little Help? Encouragement for Black Women in Ministry	Teresa L. Fry Brown	_____
Scarred by Struggle, Transformed by Hope	Joan Chittister	_____
Souls of My Young Sisters: Young Women Break Their Silence with Personal Stories That Will Change Your Life	Dawn Marie Daniels Candace Sandy	_____
Love Letters to Our Daughters: A Collection of Womanly Affirmations	Angel C. Dye	_____
All the Joy You Can Stand: 101 Sacred Power Principles for Making Joy Real in Your Life	Debrena Gandy	_____
Sacred Pampering Principles: An African-American Woman's Guide to Self-Care and Inner Renewal	Debrena Gandy	_____
The Love Lies: 10 Revelations That Will Transform Your Relationships and Enrich Your Love Life	Debrena Gandy	_____
Inner Healing for Broken Vessels: A Domestic Violence Survival Guide	Linda H. Hollies	_____
Jesus and Those Bodacious Women: Life Lessons from One Sister to Another	Linda H. Hollies	_____
Taking Back My Yesterdays: and Moving Forward with Your Life	Linda H. Hollies	_____
Don't Waste Your Pretty: The Go-to Guide for Making Smarter Decisions in Life & Love	Demetria L. Lucas	_____
Journey to the Well	Vashti McKenzie	_____
How to Avoid the Superwoman Complex: 12 Ways to Balance Mind, Body and Spirit	C. Nicole Swinner	_____
Jambalaya: The Natural Woman's Book of Personal Charms and Practical Rituals	Luisah Tesh	_____
Acts of Faith: Daily Meditations for People of Color	Iyanla Vanzant	_____
One Day My Soul Just Opened Up: 40 Days and 40 Nights Toward Spiritual Strength and Personal Growth	Iyanla Vanzant	_____
Yesterday I Cried: Celebrating the Lessons of Living and Loving	Iyanla Vanzant	_____

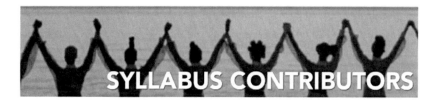

SYLLABUS CONTRIBUTORS

REV. T. DENISE ANDERSON
Pastor, Unity Presbyterian Church
Temple Hills, MD
@thesoulstepford

SUSHAMA AUSTIN-CONNOR
Program Director in Continuing Education
Princeton Theological Seminary
@sushama

REV. DR. SHELLEY D. BEST, D.MIN
President and CEO, The Conference of Churches and
The 224 EcoSpace
Adjunct Professor, Hartford Seminary
@revshelley

VALERIE BOYER
Psychology Major, Howard University
Youth Minister at Mt. Moriah Baptist Church
@womanonfire1130

REGINA N. BRADLEY, PHD
Assistant Professor of African American Literature
Armstrong State University
Nasir Jones HipHop Fellow at Harvard University
@redclayscholar

REV. VALERIE BRIDGEMAN, PH.D.
Associate Professor of Homiletics & Hebrew Bible
Methodist Theological School in Ohio
Founding President & CEO
WomanPreach! Inc.
@DrValerieB

NATALIE BULLOCK BROWN
Assistant Professor of Film and Broadcast Media
Saint Augustine's University
@nataliebb2

DR. KHALILAH L. BROWN-DEAN
Associate Professor of Political Science Quinnipiac University
Faculty Co-Coordinator, Health Policy and Advocacy Concentration
Frank H Netter School of Medicine
@KBDPHD

REV. COURTNEY BRYANT
Minister of Social Justice, Tabernacle Missionary Baptist Church
PhD Candidate Religion: Ethics and Society, Vanderbilt University
@TheWza3point0

CHERYL D. EDWARDS BUCKINGHAM
Scientist, Professor, Writer
@sourtherngyrl7

LORYN C. WILSON CARTER
Communications Strategist and Womanist
@elledub_1920

MIN. HAZEL CHERRY, M.DIV.
Faith Community, Organizer
The Expectations Project
@laydeproclaimer

MIN. CASSANDRA CLARIETT, LMSW
Licensed Master Social Worker
DMin Student, United Theological Seminary
@C_Clariett30

Chapter 3

Live a Joyful Life...On Purpose

I've coined what I'm doing now my "Ministry of Joy." Sounds a bit dramatic, but I'm convinced it's needed. I'm more and more saddened by the amount of negativity, depression and hopelessness I see in both women and men on social media, TV and in clinic. I want to encourage people to choose not just happiness, but joy. There is a difference.

Happiness is a feeling that can be fleeting, but joy is long lasting and a conscious decision and lifestyle. I'm generally a joyful person. Even when I'm sleepy or frustrated, I can muster up the energy to put a smile on my face and speak positivity into others' lives.

When I'm feeling down, I try to concentrate on doing something nice or meaningful for someone else. Seeing him or her happy makes me happier.

Bits of anxiety and depression can enter our lives at moments and overtake us if we allow it to do so. You have to wake up every day determined to find joy. I wrote the following on a recent turbulence-filled flight:

Speaking of anxiety, I'm on a plane now trying to control my nerves. We're apparently flying over some weather-related bumpiness, the pilot explains, which should calm down soon. I've never really been a fan of flying. I'm not quite to the point of needing Xanax, but I have a cocktail or two and listen to music (listening to Foreign Exchange's "Better" at the moment) to distract me. Not sure if it's working so I opened up Microsoft Word and started writing.

This weekend we attended the No Fear Ladies Conference in Oklahoma City, OK, for the first time and had a great experience. My college friend and sorority sister, Wyjuana Montgomery, did a wonderful job in her second year as the leader and hostess of this empowering event. I met Bern Nadette Stanis, better known as Thelma from "Good Times," and many other wonderful, enthusiastic women who were ready to make their next move in life. We discussed a variety of topics, but fear was at the forefront.

Wyjuana, a speaker/should be preacher (yes, I'm claiming it) in her own right, wrapped up the day's events by asking us, "Are you a grape or are you wine?" How deep this is!

The Superwoman Complex: A Follow-Up Visit

Are you content with staying where you are currently, risking stagnation, or are you ready to be picked and possibly stomped, all in an effort to be fermented and perfected, and made into a finer product? It made me think about the times I'm most afraid, now being one of them.

Anxiety can affect us in a number of ways, causing a variety of physical symptoms. Some of us feel palpitations, sweaty palms, headaches, insomnia, jumpiness in our legs, numbness/ tingling, or chest pain. Sometimes, we can use deep breathing techniques and prayer to help calm ourselves. Other times, seeking professional help and talking to your doctor or therapist is the way to go. Medications, when necessary, are helpful when combined with behavioral changes. Get the help when you need it.

But for now, while I'm on this plane, I'm going to see the metaphor in this for life. Even though life may be bumpy at times, we have to remain positive, flexible and open to change. So, I'm going to breathe easy, sit back, say a prayer (and maybe have a cocktail or two) and enjoy the ride. Onward and upward, y'all!

The best things happen when we're afraid. We usually come up with the brightest of ideas at that time. When our backs are against the wall, we can become our best. Have a Plan B, but don't give up on Plan A without trying it first. I always think back to the time I was told our clinic was being shut down and I'd have to work at a different clinic – unless my colleagues and I wanted to take over. We had zero business experience and no idea how to run a practice, but our love for our patients and community drove us to stay together, and despite the fear of failing, we joined forces to figure it out. We hired a knowledgeable management company to teach and lead us, and we're still standing six years later!

Review Questions:

1. What's my definition of happiness? What's the difference between happiness and joy to me?
2. Am I truly happy at this point in my life?
3. What can I do to create joy in my life and environment on a daily basis?
4. Am I surrounded by other happy and joyful people?

Chapter 3: Living a Joyful Life...On Purpose

Notes: _____

_____

_____

_____

_____

_____

_____

_____

_____

_____

_____

_____

_____

_____

_____

_____

_____

_____

_____

_____

_____

_____

_____

_____

_____

_____

_____

28

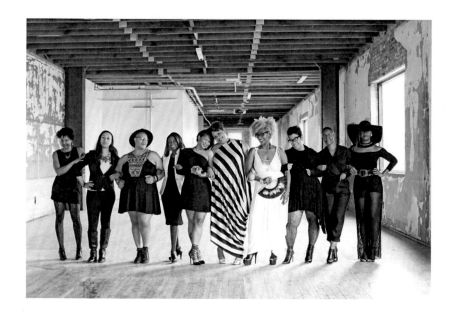

Chapter 4

Time For Your Check-Up

Taking care of yourself is an integral part of the "No Superwoman" movement. Numerous medical conditions are considered silent killers because you'd never know you had one unless a complete physical exam and lab tests revealed it. Screenings exist for that reason: to potentially catch diseases in infancy. Don't wait until you're on your deathbed to get tested for major medical conditions. Exercise preventive maintenance!

Recently, I decided to take my own advice and get an early mammogram. Though my normal breast exam, administered during a pap smear, was lump-free, my ob-gyn thought it was a reasonable idea. I also asked a good friend of mine who's an ob-gyn and the same age what she thought about getting an early mammogram, and she'd already gotten her first one. At the time, I was 37 years old with no significant family history of breast cancer, fortunately, which generally puts me at low risk. I'd also stopped birth control pills and breastfed two babies, which also puts me at low risk.

However, I was still nervous because you never know what a mammogram might reveal.

Guess what? It didn't hurt at all! I had the new and improved 3D version, which lasts a little longer but squeezes less. For my ladies who've worn really tight bras or breastfed, this was nothing. The tech that I had was lovely. I'm sure having a friendly technician to talk you through the procedure and laugh with you makes a difference. I asked her what she thought the fear was with getting mammograms, and she said it had a lot to do with a patient's anxiety level. The more afraid a woman was to get one and about what might be found, the more painful it seemed to be. She also forewarned me that since it was my first one, I would likely be called for a follow up, because there was no previous mammogram to compare it to.

I treat female patients of all ages and I've diagnosed a handful of breast cancers. Some of these women had classic or textbook risks, such as being in their late 40-60s with a family history of breast cancer, or having an abnormal lump found during an exam. However, at least two or three within the last couple of years had zero risks. One that struck me as a surprise was a patient who was healthy as a horse. She was in her 30s, didn't smoke, not on birth control and worked out all the time, but was experiencing bloody nipple discharge. As a precaution, we scheduled her for her first ultrasound and mammogram, and it was positive for cancer. I was just as astounded as she was because she looked just like me.

I've asked friends and family and the majority of them know someone in their 30s or 40s without any family history who has been affected by cancer. What has caused controversy is the recent change in recommendations for when to start and how often to conduct mammograms. Within the last five years the guidelines have changed, stating that we should wait until age 50 to begin mammograms, instead of starting at age 40, which I was accustomed to doing. Generally speaking, I would start conducting mammograms at age 40 and bring patients in for screening every other year. For those with significant family history, I would start at age 35. With the new guidelines, what happens to all of the 30 and 40 year olds we may miss? Needless to say, I've been a bit of a rebel. Maybe waiting until the early 40s is okay, but I'm definitely not waiting until age 50 to screen my patients.

Self-examination guidelines have also changed. In general, I teach all women how to examine their own breasts beginning in young adulthood. You'd think the earlier, the better applies to being comfortable with feeling your own breasts. However, with the new mammogram guidelines (USPSTF guidelines) also came the recommendation AGAINST doing self-exams. Yes, you read correctly: against. I don't feel great about that one either, but I'm a rebel with a cause and will continue advocating early intervention. Wouldn't you rather know than not know, and most importantly, sooner than later?

Review Questions:

1. When was my last physical exam, with or without a pap smear?
2. Have I ever had a mammogram?
3. When do I plan on having my first or next one?
4. Do I know if anyone in my family has a history of breast cancer? If so, at what age?

The Superwoman Complex: A Follow-Up Visit

Notes: _____

_____

_____

_____

_____

_____

_____

_____

_____

_____

_____

_____

_____

_____

_____

_____

_____

_____

_____

_____

_____

_____

_____

_____

_____

_____

_____

_____

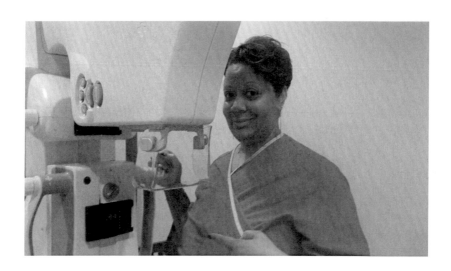

Chapter 5

The Sleepy-Mama Syndrome

The Sleepy-Mama Syndrome is a term I made up after treating a patient who's a single mother of two, works full time, takes online classes at night and is, unsurprisingly, chronically tired. We laughed about how "it just is what it is right now." But maybe things can be different.

If you know me or read the first book, you know I'm the self-appointed Nap Queen. My affinity for napping comes naturally: my father lies down for a little shuteye every day around 2 or 3pm, and wakes refreshed and ready to enjoy the rest of the day. Obviously, I can't snooze during the week because I'm at work, but hallelujah for the weekend! When the kids go down, I go down. I'm trying to pass that nap gene to them so they'll be good sleepers. Thankfully, napping doesn't affect my ability to sleep at night. Unfortunately, my hubby can't say the same. If he tries to sneak a nap in, he's up all night and tired the next day.

So, this is what we reviewed with my patient: She said she wakes up at 5am every day. Most days, she naps from 11am to 1pm (I didn't ask her how she's able to do this and work, but I will next time), gets home for dinner around 5-6pm and does homework in her bed till midnight. When she finally dozes off, she awakens again at 2am, then fights to get back to sleep until 5am. Of course, she's fatigued the next day.

She has a history of hypothyroidism, but her levels are well-controlled, so we can't blame that. Thus, I advised her to stop taking those naps for a while. She gasped and swooned at this, but I informed her that those daily naps are likely the reason she's chronically tired. Succumbing to siesta isn't beneficial to everyone. As I mentioned earlier, napping during the day leads to minimal sleep or no sleep at all for my husband. We also discussed turning off her electronics—TV, phone, computer—at least 1-2 hours before sleeping. Too much light causes over stimulation of the eyes and brain and can keep you up. Exercise is very important, and she wasn't really doing any. At least 2-3 times weekly, of at least 30 minutes is helpful for many reasons. We reviewed the rest of her medications, looking for diuretics that might keep her in the bathroom at night, or antidepressants that might keep her excited at night. We discussed her caffeine intake, making sure she didn't have any coffee or sweet tea after dinner.

Lastly and most importantly, we reviewed her stress level. She mentioned more stress than usual at work and dealing with unruly (her words, not mine) teenagers at home. We had to figure out a way to relax. Along with exercise, I suggested journaling and meditation/prayer. Over the counter, she could add some melatonin, which is a natural supplement we all have in the blood stream. It peaks in the body as bedtime approaches, so taking a little additional dose is helpful.

As mothers, we'll all have the Sleepy-Mama Syndrome at some point, some more chronically than others, but there are ways to manage the symptoms. Make sure you're aware of them!

Review Questions:

1. How many hours do I actually get every night? Do I wake up feeling rested?

2. What obstacles are in the way of me getting more sleep?

3. What are some things I could change in order to get more restful sleep?

The Superwoman Complex: A Follow-Up Visit

Notes: _____

_____

_____

_____

_____

_____

_____

_____

_____

_____

_____

_____

_____

_____

_____

_____

_____

_____

_____

_____

_____

_____

_____

_____

_____

_____

_____

_____

Superwoman Serum Body Butter

TO HELP YOU RELAX...

coconut oil, shea butter, evening primrose oil, melatonin, lavender & patchouli

amy melissa face & body & #docswiner

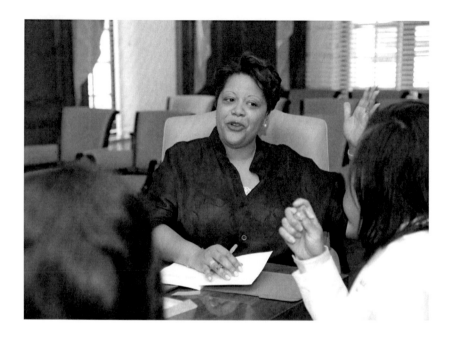

Chapter 6

The "Weight" of the World and the Curvy Controversy

I'm a little nervous about discussing this because I don't want to offend anyone. I also don't want people to look at me and say, "Wait, you're curvy!" But here goes...

Standards of beauty have loosened and society now seems to love curvy women. Many praised a popular sports magazine's feature of a plus-size supermodel on the cover, and various reality and musical stars are lauded for their "thickness." It seems we've made it a little more okay to not be paper-thin.

By social standards, I am a thick and curvy woman, and for the most part, I am very secure and confident in my appearance. However, I'm not naïve, and I'm working on being healthier. Here in the South, we celebrate curves and being voluptuous, or my favorite and most hated description: big-boned. But as a medical professional, I have to play devil's advocate. What makes me a little bit nervous about celebrating curves is the confusion it causes. For instance, I recently treated an eight-year-old patient who was majorly overweight and already had elevated sugars.

Kids are not outside running and playing as much as they used to. There is too much social media and too many electronics keeping them occupied indoors. We're eating more processed foods with too much sugar and not drinking enough water. We're working more at our cubicles, developing the dreaded cubicle booty (a wide posterior flattened from sitting on it most of the day). We're leaving sedentary jobs and going home to sit on the couch in front of the TV.

Clearly, some of us are from families that are heavier-set, which (depending on whether you believe in nature or nurture) somehow leads to most other individuals in that family being heavy. However, let me burst your bubble: All of our bones are the same size. No one is literally big-boned. Let that sink in for a moment. Have you ever seen a human skeleton either in pictures or in a lab? They're almost always the same size, aren't they? That's because they are. Generally, skeletons vary mostly in height, not weight or bone thickness.

It's not that I want you to be thin like a twig, because being skinny doesn't necessarily mean you're healthy. There are marathon runners, vegetarians and others typically considered healthy who also die from heart attacks and other diseases. We should all, no matter our weight, get our blood pressure, sugars, and cholesterol checked. If you know things are not right, there are ways you can eat better, exercise and trim down. We have to balance being proud about our curves with being healthy. If your BMI (body mass index, which factors in weight with height) is above 30%, you are officially obese. Obesity leads to diabetes, hypertension, heart disease, some cancers, and even possibly Alzheimer's dementia.

I love curvy women, but I also support you being healthy. Let's stop eating fast food and drinking sodas all the time. Stop introducing your children to sodas and processed food. And, no, diet sodas aren't always better. They have some artificial sugars that your body recognizes as real sugar. Don't have low self-esteem about your body, but keep it real and keep it healthy. Let's not settle and love yourselves to health!

Review questions:

1. Am I honestly a healthy weight? Is my BMI over 30% (which indicates obesity)?

2. Could I eat a healthier diet? What can I do today to change it if it's not healthy?

3. Am I exercising at least 2-3 times per week for at least 30 minutes at a time? If not, what could I do differently to include it in my schedule?

Chapter 6: The Curvy Controversy

Notes: _____

_____

_____

_____

_____

_____

_____

_____

_____

_____

_____

_____

_____

_____

_____

_____

_____

_____

_____

_____

_____

_____

_____

_____

_____

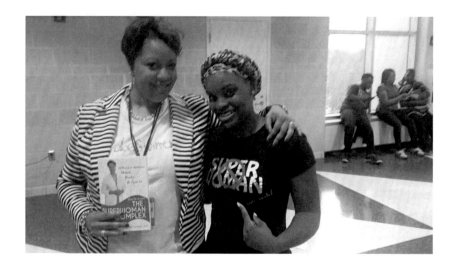

Chapter 7

Pack Light

While traveling with my family on vacation, I laughed at myself as I tried to pick up my back pack and the kids' bag all at once. I sang to myself, "Pack light..." If you're a neo-soul fan, you'll recognize this lyric from Erykah Badu's anthem, "Bag Lady." This song has been on my mind since I visited a breast cancer support group – Sisters Network – and a bright, exuberant young lady sang part of it as a way to introduce some gifts she'd brought. She lovingly distributed handmade cloth bags, using them as a metaphor for all of the "stuff" we carry around.

Before kids, I toted a nice bag of sorts, typically a shiny, new designer one. Once I had kids, my snazzy designer purse was replaced with a huge diaper bag filled with bottles, wet wipes, diapers, of course, and other things young children need. Before heading to work, I grab my computer bag and usually two other bags filled with lunch, workout attire or other stuff I think I might need during the day. The point is, we're all carrying too much.

The Superwoman Complex: A Follow-Up Visit

Without being deep, I literally mean we're carrying too much. Think of how many pounds a large bag weighs on your shoulder, neck and back. No wonder mothers deal with chronic tension headaches and muscle spasms. My favorite term is "the soccer-mom-reach-back," named for the strain put on your rotator cuffs when reaching toward the back seat to hand your child a cheerio, iPad or pacifier. We put a lot of strain and pull on those muscles over the years.

To speak metaphorically, we also carry a lot of emotional baggage. It's difficult for some of us to move on from a failed relationship, lost job or passing of a loved one. These negative experiences can drag you down longer than you realize. You think you've processed it and your feelings. You feel like you've grieved appropriately. But on the inside there's still turmoil and sadness and anger. This can be dangerous because many times, you don't recognize the effects. Very slowly and gradually, insomnia kicks in. Or comfort eating increases. Or you've suddenly become more withdrawn from the ones you love and your favorite hobbies.

But when you pack light, you let some things go. It's not easy, but you have to. Your troubles may not be so heavy, but whatever they are, be determined to get past them. Talk to someone to help you figure out what works best for you. Take a walk, write a blog or join a support group. Whatever you do, let it go.

Review questions:

1. Am I holding on to the death of a loved one or loss of a relationship? If so, why exactly?

2. From what is this holding me back? What goal can I not achieve because of carrying this load?

3. Do I need help letting go? If so, to whom can I reach out?

The Superwoman Complex: A Follow-Up Visit

Notes: _____

_____

_____

_____

_____

_____

_____

_____

_____

_____

_____

_____

_____

_____

_____

_____

_____

_____

_____

_____

_____

_____

_____

_____

_____

_____

_____

_____

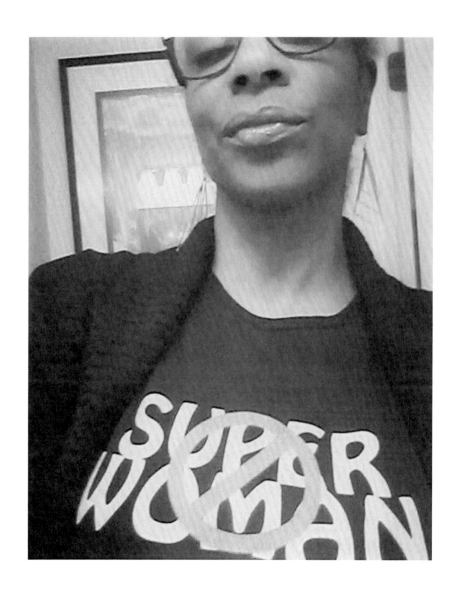

Chapter 8

Don't Rock the Boat

I'm with my husband on my first (his second) ever cruise. I was nervous, because I'd never been on one before, and I can't swim. I planned out getting a motion sickness patch, antibiotics for the possibility of Traveler's Diarrhea, and tried to prepare myself for what the feeling of the rocking boat would feel like. I planned out the days to the tee about what my girls were going to eat, play and wear, while they're staying with their Aunt.

The truth is, you can't really prepare or control for what it feels like. You just have to let go and enjoy it.

I awakened the 2nd day of the cruise and jumped onto my computer to write this. I remembered last night, feeling out of control, as the ship began to rock a little harder and sway just a little more, while I was trying to fall asleep. I looked out of our window to see the waves and wondered if we were anywhere close to the tropical storm that was near the coast of Florida, where we were traveling. I wanted to call the front desk and ask if we were close to the storm and whether the Captain was navigating around it. I later realized how silly that was and just prayed that God would calm the waters and get us through the storm. I said to myself and to the water "Peace be still" and closed my eyes to fall back to sleep.

This is a metaphor for us, Superwomen. The point is we have to let go at some point and just enjoy. The phrase "don't rock the boat" came to mind as I awakened to a much calmer morning and looked at the smoother waves outside.

Recently, in my career and business, wonderful things and opportunities have been happening. I thank the Lord that He allowed these things to come to pass, in spite of me. We often get in our own way and try to control too much. We have to remember to step out of the way and let God do what He has planned in our lives. The night before leaving for this cruise, I learned I was nominated and invited to go to the first United State of Women's Summit at the White House. I had been hoping and dreaming and applying and asking God to work this out for me. I had given up on the idea of this happening, and then all of a sudden, the acceptance letter came. I celebrated briefly, and then became fearful of HOW I was going to make it happen--- how was I going to travel; how was I going to pay for the flight so close to the event; in what hotel was I going to stay with the high cost of staying in the city, etc. Lo and behold, a dear friend of mine was already going to be in DC for work and offered for the both of us to stay together for free and drive together to be each other's company and travel with less cost. Wow! The plans worked themselves out. He let me know He was still the One in control.

So, in life, let's remind ourselves to step out of our own way and not rock the boat. We, ultimately, are not the ones in control. As a matter of fact, being a "control freak," can literally drive you crazy at times.

Have the faith that it will work out. Have the strength to speak to your situation. When things at work seem out of control, or our kids don't seem to be listening, sometimes we have to pray and let it go. When we're doing too much to control the situation, we often mess it up. Ride the waves sometimes, and just watch what happens. Enjoy the boat ride. God has your back.

Review questions:

1. What conditions in life make me the most nervous? Flying? Swimming? Changing, in general?
2. Was there something that happened when I was younger that triggered this fear?
3. How can I best deal with this fear?

The Superwoman Complex: A Follow-Up Visit

Notes: _____

_____

_____

_____

_____

_____

_____

_____

_____

_____

_____

_____

_____

_____

_____

_____

_____

_____

_____

_____

_____

_____

_____

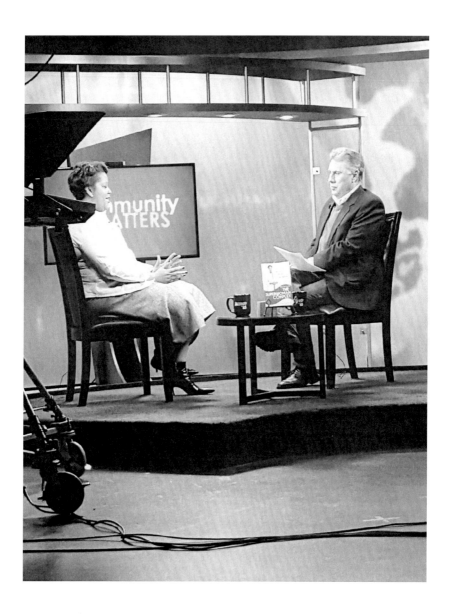

Chapter 9

The SuperMAN Complex

Let's hear it for the boys!

Since I focus so much on the ladies and women's health, I decided to show men's health some love, too. I wholeheartedly believe that some, or even more, men suffer from Superman Complex just as much as we suffer from Superwoman syndrome. Men classically and stereotypically feel the need to be heads of household, the "bring-home-the-bacon-ers" and protectors of their kingdom. Imagine the burden that must create, especially when he may not be performing or succeeding the way others think he needs to succeed.

I did a podcast with my friends and authors of the "The Makings of a Man" – O. Gerard Droze, Michael Holoman and Jabari Price – during which I answered some of their most pressing questions, and it was one of my most honest and humorous podcasts to date. Here's what we discussed:

Why is it that men are so resistant to going to the doctor in the first place?

I'm not sure why. Not sure if it's because Mom is usually always the one who made the appointments for their sons and husbands. Once they leave the home, they forget to go to the doctor. Women are in the habit of going to the doctor for their check ups a couple times a year, and men don't really go unless there is something wrong. Maybe men are afraid of what the doctor might tell them. They may feel that no news is good news. If they get sick or feel bad, it's got to be bad enough for men not to be able to function daily. If his wife doesn't schedule an appointment for him, then he probably wouldn't go.

Why is it so important for us to get a physical every year?

There are certain things that are silent killers. You don't always feel the symptoms of conditions like high blood pressure, diabetes, kidney disease. You may not know you are at risk or have these issues if you don't go to be screened for them.

How soon after the age of 40 should you have your prostate checked?

African American men after the age of 45, I believe, should get it checked. There are national recommendations through the USPSTF (United States Preventive Services Task Force) that state we should no longer check the prostate via a digital rectal exam nor do a blood test, called the PSA (prostate specific antigen). I'm a bit of a rebel when it comes to that. I will always discuss the pros and cons with each patient and almost always end up testing the PSA as a baseline for follow.

(The guys said most men are scared to go to the doctor because of rectal exams but I countered that women go through much worse. Men have the right to say, "I read that men don't always have to have a rectal exam." You can decline that and be an advocate for yourself.)

Does healthy eating impact you more than consistent exercising?
Exercise, in general, probably helps health problems more. You're working your heart, helping blood pressure, cholesterol, endorphins, etc. There are plenty of skinny unhealthy people. Once you have a good workout routine then the healthy eating should follow.

How much does stress play a part in our health?
Just about anything can be traced back to stress. My husband was a TV anchor and in sales. He was successful but his father was ill. Shortly after we got married, we were in Charleston and he had signs of gastritis. His blood pressure was very high, and we went to ER. This was without any signs of headache, blurry vision, which is why it's called a

silent killer. His stomach condition came from harboring so much stress. His job was stressful, so he decided to make a change. Are you truly happy at work? We spend a third of our day working. Who you work with, what you are working on and for how long can all cause undue stress. Take a look at your overall routine and adjust where you can. When it's time to stop, your body will tell you.

Is there anything men can do, the homeopathic way, as a natural remedy for losing their hair?
Not really. There are some over the counter products to try. If it's genetic, there's not a lot you can do without seeing your primary doctor or a dermatologist. If you feel that it's premature, I would check thyroid, vitamin and testosterone levels. Low testosterone, or "manopause" as I like to call it, is very common for men after a certain age. Both women and men go through loss of hormones with aging. I would be aware if certain things drift off, your mood, your libido, hair loss, etc. If these things start to happen, then you can always get those levels increased.

Long story short, guys, the complex can catch you, too. Don't ignore the signs and please get your check ups annually. The Superwomen can't do it without you!

Review questions:

1. Do I know a guy that may be suffering from the Superman Complex? What can I do to address this with him?
2. When's the last time a man that I care about had a physical exam and check up?
3. If I'm married to or partnered with a Superman, how can we better work together to make things easier for both of us?

Chapter 9: The SuperMAN Complex

Notes: _____

_____

_____

_____

_____

_____

_____

_____

_____

_____

_____

_____

_____

_____

_____

_____

_____

_____

_____

_____

_____

_____

_____

_____

_____

_____

_____

_____

_____

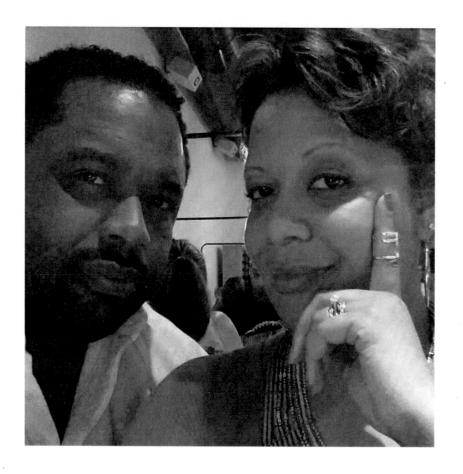

Chapter 10

How to Avoid Holiday Stress

Cheers to my favorite time of the year! This time is filled with Thanksgiving feasts and Christmas cheer, but it can also be a time of stress and overdoing. Let's get into the habit of planning ahead to make things a little easier for all of us. Here are some ideas:

1. Divide and conquer—If you're planning to get together with a large group, why not potluck it? Have a couple of key folks, the best cooks of course, bring their favorite dish to the dinner. That way, all of the pressure isn't on one particular person. Give up some of the control and share the load.

2. Delegate the duties—After the food and fellowship, divvy up household duties. Don't wait for someone to ask if you need help! Assign someone the task of bringing dishes to the kitchen, another loading the dishwasher, the trash taker-outer...you get the drift. This is especially important if you're hosting at your

house and did most of the cooking. It's only fair that the others help clean up. Even little ones can help by picking up crumbs or wiping the kids' table!

3. Clean as you go—While cooking and serving, go ahead and bring out the Tupperware and plastic wrap and start putting things in storage containers early. Don't wait until you have postprandial drowsiness (there's another common term for this I won't mention here ;-)).

4. Why cook at all? —Unless you're ultra-traditional and must have the classic layout, consider going out or ordering in. Places like Whole Foods, Harris Teeter, and other stores already have holiday foods prepared. Many enjoy buffet-style dinners or four- or five course meals at their local country club where they're served like kings and queens. Spend quality time with your friends and family instead of time cooking and cleaning!

5. A holiday "holiday"—Some of my friends are opting to spend the holidays at the beach or in a beautiful mountain cabin and eating out instead of staying home. I think it's a nice alternative. It's a change of scenery and there's less work involved.

6. Plan ahead—If you decide to cook for a large group, plan ahead and start making your recipe and grocery

lists several days beforehand. Stock up on the non-perishables and get the perishable items closer to the actual event. Utilizing grocery pick-up services is an even better idea. I pay an extra $5 for someone to grocery shop for me, schedule a pick-up time and voila, one of my biggest tasks is done! Eliminate stress by eliminating procrastination.

7. Keep it light—Was last year's holiday meal a mess because of family tension or discord? One of my patients had a major falling out with her brother at the last family gathering, the two hadn't really spoken since, and she was fearful of what the next gathering would bring. I encouraged her to call him and attempt to address it beforehand, just the two of them, so there's less of an audience, less drama and hopefully more reconciliation, resulting in a peaceful meal. Don't wait to bring up a 10-year-old argument while the turkey is being carved. It's inappropriate and highly uncomfortable for everyone else.

8. Take some "me" time—If you're hosting a family gathering, I suggest setting a side time for yourself two or three days beforehand. Get a massage, a mani/pedi or whatever relaxes you. You may not be able to afford the fanciest spa in town, but there are plenty of affordable Groupon or Living Social deals. You'll be refreshed and ready to tackle that turkey!

Review Questions:

1. Whose responsibility is it to host and plan most of the holiday get-togethers?

2. Is the work shared equally?

3. If it's usually me, would I rather share the load for this and future get-togethers?

4. Could I use one of these tactics to make things a little easier for me this year?

Chapter 10: Holiday Stress

Notes: _____

_____

_____

_____

_____

_____

_____

_____

_____

_____

_____

_____

_____

_____

_____

_____

_____

_____

_____

_____

_____

_____

_____

_____

_____

_____

_____

_____

The Superwoman Complex: A Follow-Up Visit

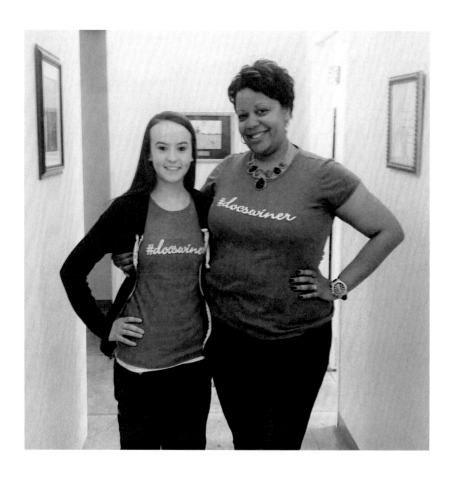

Chapter 11:

New Year, New You

This year, I created and pulled off my first women's conference, "New Year, New You 2016!" It was a hit, and I'm still on cloud 9! What a dream come true to have witnessed the ones closest to me in thought, idea and friendship come together to share this moment with me. I felt like a bride meeting her bridegroom and uniting in this light of positive energy and love. –Ok, enough waxing philosophic and let's get down to brass tax...it felt fantastic. And now, they want more!

Some pearls, to name a few, from the event were:

I spoke on the Lady Docs panel from the theme of "Do it Afraid."

Tamara Gibbs left us with the idea of a "Break Through."

Dr. Tiffany Lowe-Payne told us not forget our Faith with our medical advice.

The Superwoman Complex: A Follow-Up Visit

Wyjuana Montgomery spoke from a place of "No Fear."

We all had a similar underlying theme of keeping the faith, not giving up and living in your purpose. We spoke from places of mental/emotional/sexual abuse to a triumphant recovery.

A wonderful time was had by all, and even though I already knew what the program entailed, I was uplifted and empowered to go forward with my plans of improvement.

When I think more about "doing it afraid," I'm reminded of how this whole conference came together. I had an idea, a seed. I gathered those around me, most who are smarter and more experienced than I am, to help. I prayed about it and was steadfast, and it came together like clockwork.

Don't give up on your dream. Ask for help. Work hard and pray harder, and most things will work out.

At the end of every year, my husband and I pray together. We pray for continued protection of our marriage, household, children and health. It's particularly important to reflect on our routine, our finances and our health to see where we can improve for the next year. The goal is always a longer quantity, but more importantly, a better quality of life. We plan on what we'd like to achieve in both home and business, and then encourage one another to reach for the stars to accomplish it. Follow my journey along with me at www.docswiner.com.

So, let's all walk this scripture out this year together: "Faith without Works is Dead"–James 2:14-26. Don't just believe it; do it!

Lovingly,
Docswiner

Review Questions:

1. If I look over the last 12 months, did I accomplish all I wanted to achieve?

2. What are my new goals for this coming year?

3. What am I most afraid of jumping out there and achieving? What's one small step I can take toward achieving that goal that may not be so scary?

4. Did I like this book enough to tell someone else about it or put a nice review on Amazon? (LOL!) Then, please do!

Notes: _____

_____

_____

_____

_____

_____

_____

_____

_____

_____

_____

_____

_____

_____

_____

_____

_____

_____

_____

_____

_____

_____

_____

_____

_____

The Superwoman Complex: A Follow-Up Visit

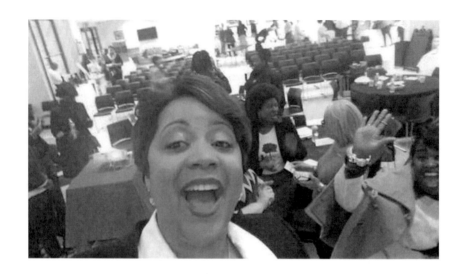

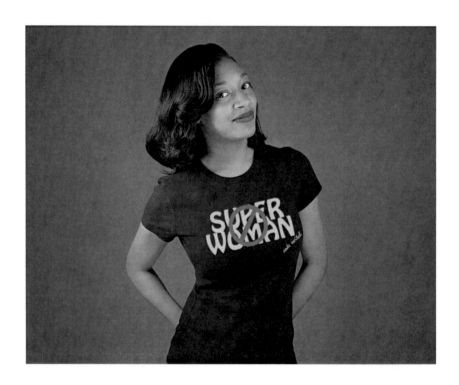

79

References

How to Avoid the Superwoman Complex: 12 Ways to Balance Mind, Body & Spirit©. C. Nicole Swiner, MD; March 2015

Lemonade Syllabus by Candice Benbow, www. candicebenbow.lemonadesyllabus; May 2016

The Makings of a Man, by O. Gerard Droze, Michael Holoman and Jabari Price; Nov. 2010

Breast Cancer Screening. USPSTF, United States Preventive Services Task Force http://www.uspreventiveservicestaskforce.org/Page/ Document/UpdateSummaryFinal/breast-cancer-screening1?ds=1&s=breast%20cancer;

Jan. 2016 Prostate Cancer Screening. USPSTF, United States Preventive Service Task Force http://www.uspreventiveservicestaskforce.org/Page/ Document/UpdateSummaryFinal/prostate-cancer screening?ds=1&s=prostate%20screening; May 2016

The Song "Bag Lady", By Artist Erykah Badu, Album Mama's Gun; 2000

Pictures

ch 1: NCCU James E. Shepard Library. March 2016

ch 2: Me and some wonderful friends in Durham. March 2016 "Lemonade" by Beyonce. Free downloadable list. May 2016. Photography by Emily Mason Photography

ch 3: Me and some wonderful friends in Durham. This time, all smiles. March 2016. Photography by Emily Mason Photography

ch 4: My first 3-D Mammogram. March 2016

ch 5: My organic sleep serum, available at https://bit.ly.docswinersstore

ch 6: My friend Mickael and I at Raleigh Women's Empowerment. April 2015

ch 7: My beautiful and majestic friend, Omi, wearing my "No Superwoman" tee. 2016

ch 8: My appearance on TV Show, "My Community Matters"

ch 9: Me and my hubby on a date night. February 2016

ch 10: Me and my friend and nurse, Jensen, at work. February 2016

ch 11: My annual Conference " New Year New You" and my shiny Superwoman tee, modeled by Tyesha. Photography by Ric Swiner Impact Imagery.